MANIFEST IT ... NOW!

Manifest It ... Now!

A 5-Step Guide to Manifesting Your Best Life

Another book from Award-winning author Dr. Christine Topjian

Christine Topjian Publishing

CONTENTS

Dedications vii

INTRODUCTION

1 - 5 Keys To Visualizing With Jesus 4

2 - How To Focus 13

3 - The Role Of Images, Visuals And Pictures . . 23

4 - The Role Of The Holy Spirit In Manifesting . . 26

5 - The Role Of The Holy Spirit In Visualizing With Jesus 38

6 - How To Be Happy While You're Waiting . . . 41

7 - "I'm Not A Believer...how Do I Do This?" . . . 48

8 - "Why Jesus? Why Do I Keep My Eyes On Him?" 50

9 - Your Calling 60

10 - Enjoy The Manifestation And Giving Gratitude 69

About The Author 77

DEDICATIONS

This book is dedicated to all those who may be struggling with either mental health issues or with being obedient and doing what God has guided them to do. May you turn to Him for strength today and always.

INTRODUCTION

Introduction:

Manifesting is powerful.

Manifesting involves a human being, charged with the power of the Holy Spirit, engaging in powerful thought processes of visualization and imagination, focusing on them, really seeing them and then powerfully applying and utilizing strong and Spirit-filled words and focus to co-create those realities with God. This will, in time and with consistent practice, lead to the manifestation (the lived reality) of what you have imagined.

We know from Genesis 1:27 that we were created in the likeness and image of God. As such, we were created to be co-creators with Christ - powerful beings who partner with Christ to bring about His best for our lives and His best timing for our lives. If we engage in prayer, Holy-Spirit-led visualizations and meditation and if we undertake strategic, Holy Spirit-led action, we become warriors in co-creating with Christ a life that is very powerful and impactful.

> If we engage in prayer, Holy-Spirit-led visualizations and meditation and if we undertake strategic, Holy Spirit-led action, we become warriors in co-creating with Christ a life that is very powerful and impactful.

"And greater works than these shall you do," is written in John 14:12. What did the Lord mean by that? It means that upon Jesus' sacrifice at Calvary, and our belief in Him, we are able to co-create an incredible life with Him, one that is beneficial to us, to society and that are Kingdom-honoring acts. Simply put: it benefits all. **Remember, nobody else is exactly you - each person is unique and the Lord has an amazing plan for each of us.** But we need to be wise enough to know about the existence of these plans and we need to learn how to tap into them.

It takes work, it takes faith and it takes wisdom (not necessarily in that order)!

Many ask the question: "Will the manifestation be immediate?" Truthfully, not likely. It takes some time for the manifestation to appear in our physical, lived reality but the wise person knows this and understands that you must wait expectantly while engaging in the practices outlined in this book which originated in Biblical teaching, because you know it will be coming.

Thank you for picking up my book. I pray that it enriches your life in Christ and your relationship with Him, allowing you to visualize, manifest and work with His best for your life.

Let's get started!

1

5 KEYS TO VISUALIZING WITH JESUS

Visualizing means seeing something in your mind's eye in a focused manner for the purposes of bringing it to your lived reality.

Allow me to explain. We all want things. Desires God has put on our hearts. We need to do certain things to access those desires. So, we need to check-in with God to see how we are supposed to access those things.

For each thing you desire, there will be different ways to access them. In other words, different steps you will need to take. But, to make this simpler, easier and more palatable, I have broken down the steps to this in 5 simple steps. They are just below.

1. Go to a quiet, distraction-free place and make yourself comfortable. Closing your eyes may help you better focus.

2. In your mind or with your mouth, ask the Holy Spirit to come into your heart and to give you a visual of what He would like to bring you. Here, you really want to let your mind go blank and clear so that you are receptive to what the Holy Spirit is bringing you.
3. The image or visual may take a moment to come or to become really clear. It is important that you recognize that this is a visual from the Holy Spirit, so you would be wise to look at all aspects of it. Ask the Holy Spirit to provide you with detailed information about what you are seeing if any part of the vision is unclear. What you will likely experience is a microscope-like "zoom-in" effect to see all that there is in a close-up manner.
4. Hold the image for some time. Really savor what you are seeing. If you get emotional, that's ok, it's not a problem (that's actually a really good thing) because that helps make the experience and the lived reality more "real".
5. When you are done looking at it, ask the Holy Spirit what you need to do to make this a lived reality. Ask the Holy Spirit to speak to you about what is required (action-wise) to make this image a fulfilled reality. When ready, ask the Holy Spirit to help you come out of the vision and then when ready, open your eyes.

Congrats! You have just visualized with the Holy Spirit!

You have taken steps toward making your best life a lived reality.

What's really interesting is that when you surrender to the Holy Spirit like this, you are really allowing the Holy Spirit to provide you with the detailed images of what God wants to bring you in real life. A comforting and happy fact is that the lived reality of this image (the physical manifestation of it) begins to happen from the moment you begin visualizing.

It is an art and a science

Visualizing is both an art and a science. It's an incredible co-creation process that we undertake to bring about anything that the Lord has put on our hearts. People all over the world have used and continue to use this method as a way to bring about God's blessings for their lives and as a means to access His best for them and for their families.

You see, science-wise, our brains cannot tell the difference between a perceived reality and a lived one. So when we see this in our mind's eye, our brains think that it is already done, so it begins to think like that and things begin to move in such a way as to bring that lived reality to your lived consciousness.

Athletes use this method to prepare for games and tournaments, business moguls use this method as a means to bring the success they desire in deal-making and in business success, single people use this to bring about meeting and marrying the love of their life, and so much more. Basically, any desire you know God has put on your heart starts to be made when you put this into practice.

Have I used this method?

You bet I have! I have visualized with the Holy Spirit and created many things and favorable circumstances, events and happenings that I have wanted to bring into my life over the years. I think back on my years of doing this and how I dedicated time to doing this (because it is work) and dedicated time to fostering the manifestation by really seeing it in my mind's eye and letting it marinate there when I have the exact picture of what I'm looking to achieve. It works every time.

It has worked in the areas of real estate, personal life, the lives of friends and family around me, matters of health, matters of deals having been materialized and money coming in and much more. I have taken the time to invite the Holy Spirit to come into my life, to help me see whatever it is He wanted to show me, to being open to what He is showing me and how it may look different from what I thought it would look like, and to giving it the time to manifest after having seen it in my mind's eye and in the eyes of my heart.

Continually working at it

Things take time to happen and to manifest in real life, so, while doing this practice one time is a good start, it does take sustained effort and doing this again and again to see real changes and sustained changes. That's why this is a **discipline**. It is something that requires daily effort of at least about 15-20 minutes per day of focused, careful visualizing, not allowing oneself to get distracted, allowing oneself to be taken to visual realms by the Holy Spirit and to really allowing ourselves to make sure that we have done all that we have needed to do on our end. After we have done all that we need to do, we need to leave it up to God to do His part because there will always be things that He can make happen that we could never have made happen on our own.

We all lead busy lives and that's fine but we all have to make sure we are investing our time into doing this and doing it right and well.

Practice

I'd like to give you an opportunity to try the 5-step process I outlined. Set aside some time today or this week and get started on this process. Remember that it is a process and we need to be mindful that any process takes a little bit of time to be accomplished. Below, I have provided some space so that you can write out what the experience was like and as you continue on this journey, you can write out what this was like the first time versus the 15th time. In this space, you can include all of the following:

- Feelings
- Ideas
- Sentiments
- Impressions
- Inklings
- Thoughts that come to you
- Words that come to you
- Sensations in your body

_____

_____

_____

_____

_____

Sensations in your body

I will talk a bit more about this point for a moment. A woman I know was happily married to her husband and shared with me her desire to have their first baby. She had wanted a baby since she was young and now that she was married and felt really ready, I advised her to try this process. She did. I advised her to be mindful of any feelings and sensations she felt in her body when she visualized. She shared that she began feeling a tummy ache when she prayed and visualized. I knew this was an indicator and told her that that seemed like a definite sensation in her body of the manifestation of this blessing and that she should keep praying and keep working on seeing it, just to be sure to complete the process until she officially took the pregnancy test and it came out positive. She did listen and found out about 3 months later that she was pregnant with their first.

What am I saying? The feelings and sensations in her body were indicators that this was going to happen. And sure enough, it did.

The time it deserves

I want to remind you that this is a process of co-creation, meaning that it is an involved process that one must respect and must learn to work with each day. That requires giving it the time it deserves and letting the steps really sink in so that you are doing it a little each day. Remember, try not to get in your own way but instead, let the Holy Spirit guide you. You may feel tempted to take over and get it done in your time frame. I caution you against this. Do this in God's timing, letting the Holy Spirit walk you through each step.

How you could feel afterwards

One piece of feedback I have gotten after giving students of varying ages time to practice this is that they felt like they were in an alternate reality but still very much in their bodies. They could actually see themselves in the eye of where the action was taking place and they were able to see other people who were integral parts of the picture, doing their parts in making things happen and moving things forward.

I remember one time when I had done this and didn't intend to (the vision came to me when I wasn't expecting it) and I was able to see every part of it. I was able to see clearly the people whom the vision was affecting (positively) and I was able to see the tears of joy from those who were happy and celebrating because the good news was going to benefit them. It was a very cool experience and I knew it was a vision because that event was not something I wanted to happen.

Community sharing

Just as you are going through things and experiencing the process, others are too. Don't hesitate to post on our community support forums at drchristinetopjian.com and let others know (anonymously if you would like) what you are going through. We were always meant to live in community and to support one another through our respective journeys and the forums on my website are intended to be a platform for just that.

2

HOW TO FOCUS

Many people find it challenging to focus when they are visualizing. Your phone can be going off, children or people can be around you, and because people may not know you are in the process of doing this, they may not know they are disturbing you. It's very simple: tell people if you need to, get yourself to a quiet space for a while, do whatever you have to do to get yourself to this quiet place and space so that you can focus on what you need to do. I liken this to having a job - a job is a place I have to go to with duties I need to perform in order to accomplish something and receive something (i.e., a blessing, compensation, etc.). This is no different. This is something you need to be mindful of and you need to train yourself to maintain focus. You can definitely also ask the Holy Spirit to help you eliminate distractions and keep your focus on the image or the mini-movie while it is happening.

Vision Boards

Another great thing to use is vision boards. Vision boards or even images pasted in your space, when done right, have all of the following benefits:

- They provide you with a visual to look at consistently, even when you are milling about the house or doing other things
- They cause you to keep the vision in your view more frequently, causing you to think about and rethink the ultimate vision
- Seeing the visuals more causes you to think about and be inspired to take the strategic action steps that will be required for the accomplishment of the vision
- They allow you to keep a Christ-honoring image in front of you, reducing the likelihood of distractions or alternatives that you may be tempted to lean towards and that would not be Christ-honoring
- The words on vision boards allow you to have specifics to look at and to read while you are working, visualizing or just going about your day
- Give you an opportunity to use words of gratitude
- Give you an opportunity to have Jesus' name front-and-center on your vision board, reminding you that these are Christ's desires for your best life
- As you are taking action and as your vision may change slightly, you can adjust your images and the words on your vision board so that certain things stick out to you more than others
- You can use the vision board to keep track of the steps required and the fulfillment and completion of a step as you are going (like a checklist)
- You can use colors and images which closely resemble what the Holy Spirit showed you so that you can keep a solid image of the visual in front of you

- As visual creatures, visuals help us conceptualize something (a picture is worth a thousand words) so you are doing your part in actively keeping the visual in front of you and actively keeping the details in front of you

It is a great idea to look at the examples of vision boards or collages that others have made, but yours needs to make sense for you. Yours needs to contain images that speak to you and that are meaningful to you. If the image does not represent what you are looking to manifest, it defeats the entire purpose of the process and it will not result in a proper manifestation.

In an effort to help you focus and keep your eyes on the proverbial prize, it's also a great idea to have words like "Believe" and "Keep the faith" and "Jesus is working on my behalf" in front of you, here and there among your living space. These words help keep you going and keep you motivated as you are journeying and doing the many things required to get going on your goals.

Actions!

After visualizing, you must take strategic, Holy Spirit-inspired actions on what you are being guided to do. For example, if you are a single person who desires to be married, visualizing is a very wise step but if you are not going to take on the actions required to manifest your marriage in the physical, then you are not fulfilling your part of the equation. You could be guided to go online to meet your future spouse, you could be guided to go to a certain party because he or she will be there, or you could be guided to do something you normally wouldn't because he or she will be present there. One of the best examples of this happened to a friend of mine who wanted to be married. She was not a Christian and I guided her to do this and she shared with me that she felt led to a particular dating app. She registered with the dating app and one by one, dismissed one guy after the next. Finally, she came across one who was not pushy, was kind and was very well educated (all things that were very important to her). The Holy Spirit guided her to take things very slowly and to build a friendship with him first because his heart had been torn to shreds and he was very sensitive. She found out by getting to know him little by little that he had been in a very bad marriage and that his wife (from whom he was divorcing) had misled him. If she had not taken things slow and taken the time to get to know him and his particular situation, she might very likely have missed out on him. To make a long story short, today she is married to him and they have two lovely, healthy and happy children.

When we visualize, we have to pay attention to the promptings of the Holy Spirit. Whether you are a Christian or not, the promptings will be there and you will get sensations, nudges and feelings that are meant to guide you to the very actions you are supposed to take. Not taking those actions will necessarily mean that you are not doing your part of the work process and therefore, you cannot blame God that He is not making something happen.

> Bottom line: We have our part to play and God has His. He will always play His part. My question is: are you playing yours?

Can I visualize and manifest the wrong thing?

This is an important question I wanted to address because the answer is yes, you can definitely manifest the wrong thing. If you do not receive an inspired word from God about something and you decide that you and you alone want to manifest something and so you spend time visualizing what you think you want, you are likely on track to manifesting the wrong thing. The manifesting I am talking about here is when we manifest based on something God has put on our heart. If you are visualizing killing someone, for example, that is not going to be something God is calling you to do.

Not getting distracted

Focus necessarily also means not getting distracted. Distractions can take many forms but the most basic definition of being distracted is that you are not doing your part in the way and in the time frame that you are supposed to. Remember earlier when I said that you have a part to play in this process and God has a part to play. He will always play His part - are you playing yours?

Here are some examples of getting distracted that you may wish to take note of. If you are guilty of not focusing, you can always pray the following prayer (in italics below the examples) to get some of the Holy Spirit's help in staying focused.

Examples of distractions:

- You know you are supposed to be completing your homework/assignment/work piece but you allow yourself to get distracted doing other more "fun" things
- You know you are supposed to be going to this event or that to meet your future spouse but you are allowing yourself to get distracted or feel lazy and not go
- You know you are supposed to reply to that really nice and proper young man or young woman you have met online that you feel the Holy Spirit guiding you toward but you are taking the time to chat with other people who may be more aggressive than them
- You know you are supposed to be working on your manuscript but at the first opportunity to go out, you jump at the opportunity and tell yourself you'll work on the manuscript another day
- You know you are supposed to be studying for your test or exam but you are using the time to go out and have fun instead
- You know you are supposed to stay home with your sick spouse but instead, you are choosing to go out with your friends and have fun, leaving your sick spouse to be home by themselves
- You know you are supposed to be working on that report for your boss because you have been aiming for that promotion but instead, you are doing other things
- You know you are supposed to be writing out and sending out the invoices to your clients for services rendered but instead, you are kicking back and watching tv, knowing that you also have payments coming up and will need that income for your own payments

Prayer to focus:

Lord Jesus, the manifestation of my desire and Your will is very important to me because I know that it will mean Your best for my life. I pray for You to help keep me focused and motivated, despite the time frames and my own impatience, and help keep me on track and doing all the things I need to do in order to fulfill what You are calling me to do and therefore, the actions and steps I need to take to bring about the physical manifestation of this blessing. In Jesus' name. Amen

Take a moment to reflect right now and think: is there anything you know you are supposed to be doing but have been procrastinating and not doing? Be honest with yourself and really think about this. If you're not sure, ask the Holy Spirit to shed some light on whether you are missing out on doing something. Write out what you are getting here. Remember, it is better to do this exercise now, while you still have time to do the action and make sure you are on His time frame and schedule.

_____
_____
_____
_____
_____
_____
_____
_____
_____
_____

It is work

I said it before and I'll say it again: manifesting is work, visualizing is work, praying is work. They are all great things to do and we are blessed to have these outlets but they are, in fact, work. They all take time, dedication and devotion. Why? Because when the manifestation does in fact materialize, it is a gift and a major blessing that you know you worked hard toward accomplishing. I don't know about you but I have not found too many gifts and blessings that manifest without a serious amount of work and doing on my part.

When we manifest, we are basically using the eyes of our heart to pray and to allow two-way communication to happen with God where we pour out our heart to Him and tell Him of our desires. He already knows but still, pouring out your heart to Him is part of the process.

When we pray, it is basically also work because when we pray, we are not only engaging in two-way conversation (prayer was always meant to be a two-way conversation) where we need to use the right words to express ourselves, but it is also the time to listen to what the Holy Spirit is saying back to us. For example, when I had just graduated Teachers College many years ago, I said this prayer out loud: "I just want to teach". Well, I did get a supply teaching job offer at a school that was quite rough, and where it was commonplace for students to throw desks, break windows, destroy technology, speak very rudely to each other and to staff, and much more. I realized from that that I needed to be much more specific with my prayer. The next time I prayed, I said this "I pray to be able to teach the following subjects at a great school very near my home and to have colleagues and students who really value me." That is a very different prayer and took a little bit of time to manifest.

This is meant to show you that your words are also extremely important. You must be mindful of what you are saying, what you are asking for and when you are making that prayer. Keeping track of when you are making the prayer helps you see the timeframe of everything involved, such as when you made the prayer, when you started visualizing, when you heard (and what you heard) from the Holy Spirit, and when you began to experience the actual physical manifestation.

3

THE ROLE OF IMAGES, VISUALS AND PICTURES

I am sometimes asked: What role do images, visuals and pictures play in manifesting? The simple answer is: a big role. The longer and more complicated answer is this: humans are visual people (we were created as visual beings) so when we have a frame of reference of a picture, an image or any kind of visual that actively represents a new reality, that is very powerful. The image can be of stick people - it doesn't matter - what matters is that it is a visual representation of a new and better reality that God wants to bring you and which you understand by looking at the image.

I remember reading an article that talked about how Kanye West wanted to marry Kim Kardashian. So, he had shared how he had taken a picture of Kim's family posing on a flight of stairs and he drew himself (as a stick person) into the image. That was a visual that worked for him. For him, it represented what he needed to visualize in order to ascertain that he was, in fact, her husband and a member of her family. Simple but powerfully effective.

When God showed Abraham the visual of all the stars in the sky, He did it to provide him with a visual of what He wanted to bring him. He knew Abraham and knew what visual would work for him, and it did. In the same way, God knows you better than you know yourself, so when He gives you a visual or invites you to select a visual for blessings He wants to bring you, He is in fact guiding you to make that reality more solid and anchored in your life, causing it to come into your life more fully and wholly.

God gave me a visual that was unmistakably clear for me in terms of something He wanted to bring me. I have 0 drawing ability so I replicated what I saw in my mind with little stick people. It was a very simple but very powerful visual that I used for days in an effort to let that visual really stick in my mind and to wrap my head around what God wanted to bring me. Next to it, I included little words and short phrases that indicated the main messages and that would help in making the visual much more concrete and understandable to me. In my book, Manifest It!, I talk a lot about vision boards and their effectiveness. They are a very effective tool and one that we are invited to use to help us frame what is to come and to help us really understand the vision and all it comes with. One of the most interesting things is that as you move through life and experiences, you can continually tweak the image you created and the photo to reflect new little add-ons.

For example, I was looking to publish a certain number of books (which, at the time, I thought was a lot), and then I read about a very famous and well-known author who has published 10 times that number and made them all quality pieces of literature. I began to wrap my head around the fact that I can do better than the original number I wrote. It pushed me not only to set my sights higher and to consult with the Holy Spirit for how many books God was calling me to write, but also prompted me to consult with the Holy Spirit and to see how I should make a plan for how I was going to publish way more than I had originally thought to do and set out to do.

This is also an important life lesson: who you keep around you will influence how far you will go in life and what you will do in life. If I hadn't been a faith-filled person, I likely would have thought that just publishing a couple of books and making that my end game literature-wise would have been sufficient. Instead, I have in my environment (inside of me) One who is pushing me to far greater.

When we step away from our visual even for a little while and then revisit it after a time, we can look more carefully with fresh eyes and we can re-examine the image with a greater focus, enhanced perception and with a renewed perspective. My image for my first books looks nothing like my image for my next and subsequent books. I am much happier with the new image and feel it is much more developed, more carefully thought-out and much more reflective of the person I am now. We change as we move through life - why shouldn't our images? The images God gives you will change as you move through life and as you continue your walk with Him.

4

THE ROLE OF THE HOLY SPIRIT IN MANIFESTING

Ultimately, it is God through the Holy Spirit who gives us the visual and who makes anything manifest for us. It is the Holy Spirit who aids us in making the manifestation happen by giving us the visual and its details and will inspire us on what actions to take.

When we realize that "this needs to be done" - that's the Holy Spirit guiding us.

When we ask a question of the Holy Spirit and we feel the sensation of a response, that is Him guiding us and assisting us.

The Holy Spirit is one of the three entities of God.

The following is a diagram that may help with this understanding.

Father (Father God) ――――――――――> Son (Jesus, who is also God) ――――――――――> Holy Spirit (Entity Spirit that lives in us when we are baptized and that acts as our Helper, our Counselor, our Truth-teller)

The Holy Spirit is basically God residing within us and being our Helper, our Truth-teller, and our Guide. He is the One who causes the thing to manifest. The Holy Spirit is the Truth-Teller, guiding you to the right understanding, actions, and thought processes you need to achieve and to manifest. The world could be telling you to do X but if the Holy Spirit is guiding you to Y, then please go to Y.

Here are 3 examples that others have experienced that showed them the steps required when they visualized. These are the steps they felt inspired (through the Holy Spirit) to undertake.

1. Deanna felt inspired to take action and write her first comic book. She always knew she would be a writer but didn't have any relationship with God so she didn't know anything about visualizing. She applied the 5-step process I have outlined in this book and slowly, she began to sense a prompt that she should write a first draft of her first book with very rough sketches. She was a bit perplexed that she was being led to write a comic book because she didn't feel that she had any drawing or such artistic abilities. But, she prayed for help with this and felt led to a drawing class. Within a few months, she began drawing her characters beautifully and finding her

artistic voice. She really enjoyed the process. She realized that she had been paralyzed in her drawing abilities because of an offhand, unkind comment a teacher had made to her many years ago about her art and since then, she didn't feel she had the confidence to create her drawings properly. Then, she felt led to an art school where she met an instructor who was also publishing these works on the side. She prayed about publishing with him and sure enough, the Holy Spirit was encouraging her to do this. Deanna's life began changing step by step and she was very grateful for all the changes. One she began making money from her comics, she was over the moon happy and grateful. She knew that she was being guided by the Holy Spirit each step of the way, which she found amazing because really simply, she did not consider herself a Christian person. She had long considered herself an atheist. As her gratitude piece, she decided to donate some of the proceeds from her book sales to a local art school to help other students who may not have the necessary financial resources to pay for the class.

2. Roger was in a really unhappy marriage and didn't consider himself a person of faith. He was not interested in visualizing for a long time until a friend of his encouraged him to do it and showed him how he had visualized better things for himself. Roger seemed to relent and be willing to give it a try. He began very small and only wanted to spend about 5 minutes per day doing this practice. Even so, he proceeded and within about a month, he began to see major shifts happening. He then began doing this practice for about 15 minutes per day and began to see how major shifts were starting to take place within him, and he began to feel himself being led to take this action or that one. He began to feel inspired by the Holy Spirit

and began to get a sense of how this works and how this needs to be done. He shared that because his marriage was an unhappy one, that he had felt unhappy and angry with God for bringing him this woman, but we talked about things and we began to see how due in part to his lack of a relationship with God, that he had been misguided into marrying this particular lady. Roger began to see how this process was starting to improve his life. He was elated when he began to see good things manifesting for him and as a result, he decided he wanted to start a gratitude writeup and blog.

3. Joey worked hard each day to provide for his family. He was a hard worker but felt something significant was missing. He had been raised in church but was not at all aware of manifesting and how to engage in Spirit-led visualizations. He was not at all aware how he could apply this to better his life and to allow to manifest what God wanted to bring to him. He began to engage in this process and for a little while, he felt that nothing significant was happening. He began to feel discouraged and he had to pray many times for the courage and the motivation to undertake this process. He went to the doctor and found out that he was sick and that recovery was going to take some time but that there was a cure for the illness. He was not at all happy but he knew that he needed to stay strong for the sake of his family. He did. We prayed together over this and he began to be open to the possibility of visualizing. He felt he was being given a vision of great health and that this ailment was behind him. He felt that the Holy Spirit was communicating that he would be over this illness and return to great health. I encouraged him to listen carefully to the promptings and to do as he was being guided. I reminded him that even

little inklings are a communication that must be listened to. He began to pick up his old university medical textbooks that he had long ago abandoned. Joey was a premed in university but left school because his father had passed away and he felt he needed to work full time to provide for his family. He had left school and a promising career as a doctor in order to work full time and be there for his family after such an important passing. He began to pick up his books again and felt such an ease and facility with the textbook material but he knew he didn't have the funds to go back to school. The Holy Spirit was leading him to apply for a scholarship because his grades were really quite good. But, the scholarship applications required recommendations from past professors, and it had been a long time since he had been in school. He didn't have what was required of him. I encouraged him to press into the vision and to seek the Holy Spirit's answer on this. Joey contacted one of his former professors and asked him if he would, after all this time, provide him with a reference. The prof immediately agreed and told him he had incredible promise and that he admired what Joey did to provide for his family. Everything was starting to line up. Joey submitted his scholarship applications and was granted a partial scholarship. He then felt led to apply for a special bursary for students who are first generation immigrants, which he was. The two scholarships together were enough for his entire tuition and he went back to school, while also working as a TA (teacher's assistant) to make some additional money, in addition to a part time night job he got online to help pay the bills. His family members also were now old enough to work and so they helped out a fair bit, allowing him to rest a bit more easily about the family finances. Joey's life was changing and getting better the more he was engaging in this practice and following God.

God is always looking to give us His best. He is always looking to give us the best He has and always wants to make sure that we are following Him so that He can lead us and guide us to His best. Just as He gave Abraham the vision of the stars in the sky (which was way more than Abraham had asked for), He wants to do the same for you.

We have ideas about what we would like but it isn't until you take it to God that you will have an invaluable partnership with Him and frankly, you and I and everyone else needs Him to bring those good things to come to pass for their lives. He wants to bring these things to you and has given us the tools to bring these things to come to pass. He has given us the guidebook manual - are you going to use it?

The world vs. the Holy Spirit

This is a very important point. The Holy Spirit is God's provided Helper who resides within us following baptism. He literally is a Spirit who lives within us and is our Guide, our Helper, our Truth-Teller, and our Compass. He is the One who shows us the truth when the world could be telling us something incorrect or misleading, even if it is said to us with good intent. People don't know what God knows and so following people (if it is contrary to what God is saying) is not the wisest course of action. When something doesn't seem right or feel right to you, that is the Holy Spirit trying to talk to you and bring your attention to something that isn't right so you can do something about it. Anytime we ignore the promptings of the Holy Spirit, we are working against ourselves for God's best and that's just not very smart.

> Work with God because He is working for your best.

The unfortunate fact is that the world and the people in it won't necessarily always tell you the truth. People can lie, can deceive, can cover things up, for one reason or another. So, when the Holy Spirit is telling you something different from what others are telling you, you would be wise to listen, to pay attention and to go the way the Holy Spirit is telling you to go.

People also like to talk things out. People need help and understanding and to vent their ideas, thoughts and frustrations out. Especially since the start of the covid pandemic, mental health needs have spun out of control and people need to have an outlet to express themselves, no matter what they are going through. Talk to God about it. Unload it onto Him because nobody cares for you more, is more available for you and loves you more than He. Your friends and family may mean very well but they do not have the same capacity that God has to listen, to be there, to guide and to shift things in your favor at all hours.

I always say the two following points:

1. Whether it's 2 am or 2 pm, the Holy Spirit is there to listen, to talk to you, to counsel you, and to tell you the truth about anything you are dealing with
2. When the world is guiding you to X direction but the Holy Spirit is guiding you to Y direction, listen to the Holy Spirit and go the way He is guiding.

The Holy Spirit is part of God and so, has the mind of God. He can see 360 degrees, knows what is happening because He is Omnipresent and Omniscient and is already in the future, so if He is telling you to be careful, heed that warning. If He is telling you to move forward on something, you would be wise to ask how and then do so. If He is telling you that something is not for you, as great as it seems, respect that because that thing isn't but He will bring you better for you. A recent example comes to mind: I was about to accept a work offer that sounded wonderful. It seemed perfect for me, but the Holy Spirit was telling me to stay away from it. It made no sense to me. It seemed like a perfect offer to me and I was very excited about it. Instead of leaping forward, I decided to pray over it and it was clear that the answer was a no. But, as we humans sometimes do, I chose to go my own way and decided to give the job a shot, thinking that I'm sure it was going to be fine. Boy do I wish I had listened to the promptings to stay away! That job was one of the worst experiences of my life: the people managing were exceptionally rude, we were all being mistreated and told (not asked) to do things that were completely unacceptable while we were treated very poorly, being disrespected at every turn. In hindsight, I can see why the Holy Spirit was guiding me to stay FAR away from it but as we sometimes do, I went my own way and realized too late that I had made the wrong decision. Whenever those instances happen to me, it serves as a great reminder that I should have (again) listened to the promptings.

Another example is when I was interested in a particular man many years ago. The Holy Spirit was clearly telling me to stay away from him and that he wasn't the right person for me - that he is meant for someone else. I chose not to listen and I went ahead and paid attention to him, spent time with him and flirted with him. As I got closer to him, the warning was getting louder until finally, he got together with someone else and I got slammed emotionally as a result. There were signs and clues all along but I chose to ignore them. I hope you, reader, don't do that.

The Holy Spirit manifests

To be clear, you and I do not manifest. Manifestation comes from the Holy Spirit and happens in God's way and in God's timing. Our role in the process is the following:

1. Get to a quiet place and focus on visualizing. Focus the eyes of your heart on Jesus.
2. Ask the Holy Spirit to give you a visual of what He wants to bring you
3. Pray based on the promptings of the Holy Spirit
4. Meditate on the images with the help of the Holy Spirit
5. Ask the Holy Spirit questions, questions and more questions about the images and about anything else you want to know

6. Take inspired actions based on the guidance of the Holy Spirit and in the timing provided by the Holy Spirit

Timing

The timing provided by the Holy Spirit is very important. When you are provided with instructions for actions to take, there is a time frame that is very important and must be adhered to. What I mean by that is that if you are being prompted to do something within a window of time, not doing it within that window is going to delay everything and you won't get the fullness of what you are supposed to get because you didn't follow the timeline provided. The timing of things is extremely important and you are advised not to ignore the time window. God is setting things up for you within a certain frame of time and not complying with that is going to mess things up.

I liken this to putting in an application for something. There is a stated deadline and you must adhere to it. If you get your application in after the deadline, your application may be totally complete and well-written - you got it in too late and therefore, it will not be considered. This is not very smart. It's the same here. When God gives you a time frame, respect it and work within it. Anything outside of that time frame will not be helpful and will likely not be considered.

Also, adhering to timelines is a sign of respect. You are respecting God's organization, timelines, and processes. I liken this to applying to work for an organization or applying for anything: each organization has their set timelines and deadlines and if you don't get things in by the due dates, it is a pretty clear sign that you are not willing to work within their processes and then, frankly, why would they take you on?

I also want to make it clear that the manifestation of your desire may not look exactly as you think it will nor might it happen in the time frame you would like. It will likely look a bit different and that's not a bad thing. As humans, we tend to want instant gratification and that's just not God's way. God's way is to take His time, plan it out carefully, communicate it to you carefully through the Holy Spirit, be available for questions, and then help you execute it at the right time and in the right ways. Think of the manifestation of your desire as a surprise that God wants to bring you. He has wrapped it with nice wrapping paper, tied it with a really lovely bow and your name is on it so when you open it, He looks forward to it being a happy and welcome surprise for you.

One of the manifestations of my desires happened on a lazy Sunday afternoon, while I was checking my emails. I had received a surprise email from a man from my past who still meant a great deal to me. Getting his email was a total surprise and his words were sweet, kind and thoughtful. At the time, I didn't immediately recognize it as a manifestation of what I had been asking for because I didn't know the purpose of this man's email to me but as time went on and I could see his shyness, sweetness and the select words he was using to communicate what he wanted, I was beginning to see and understand his sweet and gentle approach. It was a real surprise and I was not in any way expecting it.

"How can I be sure it's the Holy Spirit?" many ask.

This is a very important question and one that is imperative to ask. Deception may come and so it's very important to qualify the source of the message or the opportunity. As such, we need to consult with the Holy Spirit to find out the authenticity of a message or a vision. The Holy Spirit is known as the Truthteller for a reason. He is the One who will tell us whether the message we are receiving is genuinely from Jesus or if it is not.

He will speak to your heart and He will tell you if it's really from Him. It is also very helpful and biblical to have advisors who are of the Christian faith. Advisors can be former teachers or professors, members of the clergy, a friend who is a Christian, etc. These are people who will help you in discerning the source of the message and who will be there to help you understand the message.

5

THE ROLE OF THE HOLY SPIRIT IN VISUALIZING WITH JESUS

When we visualize the way God intended, know that we are relying on the Holy Spirit to be our Guide. This is a significant advantage to just visualizing on our own. On our own, as mere humans, we can rely on our own strength and abilities but that wouldn't be the wisest way, especially when we have the Holy Spirit there, available, ready and willing to help us. When we visualize and pray and rely on the Holy Spirit through Jesus, we are accomplishing things in God's strength, which is obviously much more powerful than our own. Much more.

The Holy Spirit is the One who works on our behalf, providing guidance, clues and cues to help us with our manifestation journey. It is His role to provide us with the strength as well when we are looking to visualize because really simply, life can get to be very challenging and we need to be relying not on our own strength to accomplish things.

As soon as you visualize, the Holy Spirit gets to work actively on our behalf, causing events, people and circumstances to shift and to move so that everything is set up for the manifestation to occur. As soon as you visualize or pray, the Holy Spirit gets to work actively on our behalf to move out of the way people who oppose us and oppose God's plans for us. As soon as you visualize, the Holy Spirit begins to influence the right people, scenarios and situations to make things happen for us.

When we pray genuine prayers, we are humbling ourselves and telling God that we need Him, we need His strength, we need Him to do the things that we cannot do and as such, He begins to move things on our behalf and within our best interests. This is such an important thing to happen for us because if I can have the strongest Entity in the world working behind the scenes for me, why would I not want that?

Here is a suggested prayer you can use to help make things happen in your favor and in God's strength:

Lord Jesus, thank You for the words provided in this book, which help to open my eyes to all the good works You can, have, are and will do in my life. I pray that You not only help me visualize and pray based on Your will and for my benefit and the benefit of the greater good, but that the Holy Spirit comes alive inside of me and shows me how to take strategic actions in the ways that You know need to be done. In Jesus' name. Amen

After you have prayed this prayer (or some version of it that you feel compelled to), sit back, pay attention to any promptings and wait for Him to communicate next things to you. He has started working on your behalf so the instructions may be to just wait. People sometimes think that after praying, things will happen immediately, within seconds or minutes. That is not often the case. While we do know that He will cause things to happen for us, we do have to wait and be patient for things to happen in good timing.

6

HOW TO BE HAPPY WHILE YOU'RE WAITING

This is a very important point. We have prayed. We have visualized. We have done all that we felt prompted to do. Now, how do we wait while being happy and in good cheer? Simple. There are a variety of things you can do to help you wait in good cheer. Here are just a few:

- Take a nice long walk
- Listen to calming music
- Bake or cook something in the kitchen
- Do a workout
- Write out the things you already have in your gratitude journal
- Go watch something fun and funny on television or via a streaming platform you use
- Go volunteer and do good unto others
- Put in extra time at work
- Work on your hobby(ies)

- Be of service to others in need (ex. Meals on Wheels, shelters, etc.)
- Take a nice long shower or bubble bath
- Get a mani/pedi
- Read a great book or article(s)
- Catch up on your emails or correspondence
- Do something that makes you feel good, like a massage
- Congratulate yourself for undertaking this challenge (that not everyone out there does)
- Play with your pet
- Buy yourself flowers or tickets to a great sporting event or show
- Watch some comedy shows or comedy stand-up to help get you into the laughing mood

 Take a few moments right now and jot down the ones you feel you would like to do or add your own to the list and write them down in the space provided. Remember that when you write it down, write it somewhere where you are going to see it again, you are going to refer back to it and you can make tweaks and modifications to it if need be. As you grow, your ideals are also going to change and this list will change. Keeping the original is handy so you can see how you have changed over the years as well.

_____
_____
_____
_____
_____

Working out and mental health

When we are waiting for our blessing to manifest, we can get caught up in worry and we can begin to feel depressed. A great and proven way to combat that is by working out and doing yoga. Working out and yoga provide great outlets for our bodies to get into movement, to get the internal blood flowing and cause our bodies to have oxygenated blood running through our systems, and can contribute to weight loss, which will mean that you will look better and more fit and lean. All bonuses!

People who feel depressed more frequently are those who work out less and don't get into the habit of movement. You do not have to run like an Olympic runner to get the benefits I am describing here - even a short walk at a brisk-ish pace would be a great mental health boost.

In sum, don't get caught up in getting stressed and nervous about the waiting process. Instead, help yourself by engaging in other activities which will allow you to feel better and keep busy during the waiting process.

 Take this opportunity to write out the things you would like to do which you believe can be great stress relievers. If ideas are not free-flowing, ask a friend who knows you well to help you with this list. They can jog your memory about what has helped you in the past and what works well for you.

_____
_____
_____
_____
_____
_____
_____
_____
_____
_____
_____
___

Who are your friends?

Who we surround ourselves with and spend time with are very important. Our friends, acquaintances, family and surrounding environment greatly influence us in ways that we may not initially understand or take stock of. When we surround ourselves with people who speak negatively, who are always down on themselves, who constantly see the proverbial glass as half empty, who never work out or take care of their mental, emotional or physical lives, who don't take care of their finances, and much more, we can begin to consciously or subconsciously be influenced by that...and not to our benefit. You have a much higher chance of experiencing success when you are around people who are motivated, positive, go-getters and more.

I recall having a co-worker who was always so negative. She would always speak terribly over her life, would refuse to work out (even to go for a walk), would eat just terribly because she claimed that no foods agreed with her system, and more. I suggested a myriad of ways to help her but she was not having any of it. She had reached a point in her life where she was comfortable being miserable and no amount of talking, motivating or encouraging on my part or on the part of others around her was going to change her mind. She had been in this state for years and simply refused to do anything to help herself.

Simply put and this point was stated earlier in the book but is so important it bears repeating: who we have around us and who we choose to spend time with will have a tremendous influence and impact on us. Choose the people who surround you very carefully, especially while you are in your waiting period. They can bring you up and allow you to feel hopeful and optimistic or they can bring you down and cause you to sink into depression. Ask the Holy Spirit to help you select who the right people are for you and whom you should keep in your life.

7

"I'M NOT A BELIEVER....HOW DO I DO THIS?"

Many people who are unsure if God exists or who are outright atheists ask me this question. My simple answer is to try it and see what happens. God always answers. He seeks us and has chosen each of us to be in relationship with Him. Even if you are not a believer today, it doesn't mean that you can't come to Him and ask Him to show you who He is.

Ask Him to come into your life and to show you who He is. Ask Him to show you what blessings He wants to bring you.

One thing I caution people who are not believers is the following: if someone has done you wrong (even a clergy member in a Church or Parish somewhere), do not extrapolate that and pin their misdeeds on God. Many in Churches and Parishes do not do what they are supposed to and I take no pleasure in saying that. They don't treat people correctly and they sometimes don't take the time to think carefully about how they speak to people or treat people. Don't let that previous experience turn you off from your own relationship with God. Your relationship with Him is special, important and very unique. God, Jesus and the Holy Spirit are not the same as people.

8

"WHY JESUS? WHY DO I KEEP MY EYES ON HIM?"

Many people may ask "Why should I keep my eyes on Jesus?"

It's a fair question. Some who don't know Him or don't know Him well or even some who feel they do know Him but are still not sure of the answer to this may feel the need to ask this question.

Jesus is the One who has been given all authority on earth and in heaven. This means that nothing happens without Him and without Him knowing about it and approving it. Nothing. Some then may ask "Well, does He cause bad things to happen to people?" No, He doesn't. But He sometimes allows some bad things to happen but it is always for a good reason: to teach people a valuable lesson and to be right there with them and for them while they are in the thick of it.

To give an example of how the Lord intends good to come out of a bad situation, a friend of mine was dealing with a cancer diagnosis in their family. Of course, the entire family was devastated and they chose to band together, and to work together at helping the person pull through. They each began doing something that would bring the family together in a fun way: one began hosting a Friday night ritual of watching comedy movies and laughing together as a family, another began hosting a Sunday afternoon bbq where they could all get together and spend time in joy, another chose to drive the loved one to the hospital for their treatments and on the way, would play soothing, classical music. They all chose to do something to support and to inject happiness into their loved one's day. They banded together and they explained to me how they were doing what they could to keep the happy mood going and not to ever dwell on the disease. They never once referred to their family member as being sick but instead, they thanked God that the family member was well, totally healthy and spoke and acted as though the person had already beat the disease.

In Matthew 28:18, we are advised that all authority in Heaven and on earth have been given to Jesus. Since He is the One who governs everything, He is the One who will allow both good and bad things to happen. He does not do this because He doesn't love us. Good parents and guardians do not reprimand or correct a child in an effort to be nasty or horrible to them. They gently reprimand and correct because they love them and therefore, want to help them realize right from wrong and so they help them by correcting things when they are wrong. Ultimately, He is the One who approves and runs things, so to speak, but He doesn't intend these things to be a means to destroy us. Instead, as a means to teach us good values and to lean on Him and rely on Him. As such, when we would like good things to come and we are looking for blessings, for help, for breakthroughs, for success - we need to learn to look to Him.

Keep in mind, sometimes, things may seem good on the outside. The appearance may look good and may seem appealing but inside (when you look more closely), it is deceptive because it really isn't so good.

I will provide an example that happened to me. I had a space that I needed to rent and I received a rental application from some people. On paper, they seemed amazing. Polite, kind, courteous, considerate and more. If anyone reading this knows how real estate works, we tend to rely heavily on credit scores and such - they had great credit scores. On paper, everything seemed great, so I signed the lease document. Then, after they got the keys, they reneged on many of the points we had agreed upon. They made my life a living hell and refused to comply with the rules. As time went on, I could see how my faith was being tested along with my patience. But I also remembered to lean on Him and to rely on Him to get me out of the problem. Now, I know that I am not the only person to whom this has happened. People everyday deal with things that need to be managed, things that don't go as planned, things that pose a problem, a difficulty or a challenge and much more. I also know that I am not the only one who has to lean on Him and rely on Him. I have to do this daily, sometimes a few times per day.

The same holds true for blessings and for manifesting good things. Good things come from Him and He is instructing us, through Biblical stories, how He brought blessings to the people in the Bible - He can and will bring them for us too.

It is also important to pay attention to the instructions of the specific steps we need to take in order to access those good things. Everything requires action. We can have all the faith in the world but if we don't get up and work, we will not make money. We can have all the faith in the world but if we don't take care of our bodies and our minds, we are not going to feel good. We can have all the faith in the world but if we don't treat our relationships as the important, active, living and vibrant things they are, we are not going to enjoy happy and successful relationships.

Counting on things manifesting is no different. There are specific actions that need to be taken (I covered them in the first chapter) and if we don't do those things on a regular basis, we are not going to access our blessings.

Reflection time: I'd like to give you an opportunity right now to think about whether you rely on Jesus. Do you believe that He is the One who will bring you the good things you desire and will cause good things to manifest for you? Ask yourself these questions earnestly and see what you believe the answer to be. If you do rely on Him, give yourself some detailed examples of how you have relied on Him. If you don't, consider praying about how you can and should rely on Him (more). Use the space provided below to write out your responses. Remember that if you need more space, to take a journal and jot down much more. It's always a good idea to keep these responses in a safe place so you can come back to them later and you can see how far you have come and how your responses change over time:

_____
_____
_____
_____
_____
_____

Reflection time action steps:

Take another moment right now and think about your goals and dreams. When you visualize them, what does the Holy Spirit speak to you and guide you to do (action-wise) to achieve those things? What do you feel led to do in order to achieve the things God has put on your heart? Are you being led to call someone? To email someone? To set up a meeting with someone? Do you need to ask God to open a certain door that you need opened and know that only He can open this door? Do you need to refrain from doing something in order to cause that door to close so that another can open?

Pray, meditate and write out your thoughts and directions here: (Remember, the more detail you put in this now will help better and more carefully guide your next steps).

_____
_____
_____
_____
_____

Sometimes....a door has to close

This is a really important point and I wanted to give it a little more attention in this chapter. Sometimes, God calls us to close the door. He has better for us and so He guides us to be strong and to close the door in faith, so that He may bring us better. Here are some examples:

- Close the door on a previous relationship so that He can bring you the person that He has created for you
- Close the door on a previous friendship that is guiding you the wrong way so that He can bring you better (or into closer relationship with Him)
- Turn down that job that He has told you is not right for you so that He can bring you the right one
- Let go of that previous hope you were holding onto because He has spoken to your heart and told you that there is better for you
- Let go of getting into that school because He has spoken to your heart and has told you He will get you into the right school and the right program at that school
- Let go of that previously-loved one who is no longer around so that He can bring you a new beginning

God does not close a door without opening another. If He has asked you to close a door, it is because He has something better for you and in time and in faith, He will bring that to you.

I recall how the Lord had told me that I was going to need to leave my employer. I had been working there for quite some time and really didn't know much else. I wasn't sure what else He was guiding me to (I had a feeling but I was definitely not sure) so this was a big step for me and I wasn't yet sure it was a step I wanted to take. Time after time that I went to work, I sensed that He was telling me that this was not right, that I was not going to continue with this. It began to get to the point where I was wondering why I was feeling so unhappy and why I felt like I was being punished. He reminded me in my spirit that He had guided me not to take that work anymore - but I was continuing anyway. It came to the point where I had to take a firm stand and I had to walk away, remaining focused not on the door that was closing, but on the new door that needed to be opened. Sometimes it takes a big "gulp" when you're doing it and you need to pray for the courage to do it and do it right. So, if that's you, gulp away and do it. Staying on the wrong path that He has guided you to close will not ultimately benefit you.

Ask yourself: "Is there a door God is asking me (and maybe has been asking me to close for some time now?)

Write out your answer here:_____
_____
_____
_____
_____
_____
_____
_____

59

9

YOUR CALLING

This is one of my favorite topics. Your calling. Each person has one (and often, more than one). This is the very thing you are being called to do and do well because you are the only one who can do it quite like you.

The one who tells you what your calling is is God. He created you and He is the One who can show you the skills and the amazing talents you have within you that will allow you to do all that you need to do within that calling. For some, it's police work, for others, it's teaching or writing or acting or designing clothes, or designing rooms or spaces, for some others it's understanding how a vehicle engine is supposed to work and making it work the way it's supposed to. But one thing I learned is that most of the time, just because we have a calling, it does not mean that the door will just magically and amazingly open. Sometimes it's quite the contrary. When I was first getting involved in writing books, the doors certainly weren't flying right open for me. I had to put in countless hours, sending query letters, working hard at making sure my manuscript and my submissions to publishers were up to snuff, and much more. And door after door slammed (not gently closed) in my face. Nevertheless, like so many of you, I had to persevere and keep going. I had to keep on....well, keeping on. I needed to find the way that made sense for me, so I started my own publishing house where I could publish my books and the books of others I thought would be great to add to the collection. Ultimately, as is with any other person's calling, He invites you to do something because nobody else will do it quite like you. I know that I have a good eye for books and for quality literature so if I am being led to do this, then I know there are wonderful literary works He wants me to bring to market.

Just start

The old adage says it's best to start with something. If you're a filmmaker, grab your cell phone and start shooting something. If you're a writer, start by writing something. If you're a mechanic, start by fixing and repairing your friends' and family's cars. Start where you are and you will see how it all grows and expands. You will see how God will slowly start to pull back the curtain and He will begin to show you the path that He has for you. Taking it a step further, let the Holy Spirit show you what He wants you to see.

Let's apply the 5 step process here that we outlined.

1. Go to a quiet, distraction-free place and make yourself comfortable. Closing your eyes may help you better focus.
2. In your mind, ask the Holy Spirit to come into your heart and to give you a visual of what He would like to bring you. Here, you really want to let your mind go blank and clear so that you are receptive to what the Holy Spirit is bringing you.

3. The image or visual may take a moment to come or to become really clear. It is important that you recognize that this is a visual from the Holy Spirit, so you would be wise to look at all aspects of it. Ask the Holy Spirit to provide you with detailed information about what you are seeing if any part of the vision is unclear. What you will likely experience is a microscope-like "zoom-in" effect to see all that there is.
4. Hold the image for some time. Really savor what you are seeing. If you get emotional, that's ok, it's not a problem (that's actually a really good thing) because that helps make the experience and the lived reality more "real".
5. When you are done looking at it, ask the Holy Spirit to help you come out of the vision and then when ready, open your eyes. Take a moment or two to come to and jot down your take-away(s) from this experience.

When you are writing down your take-aways, make sure that you write out in detail your impressions, visuals, images, nudges and anything else you feel is relevant. Remember that the Holy Spirit speaks in a variety of ways so jot down everything, even if it doesn't seem relevant right now and you can always pray and seek clarification for something afterward.

Impressions jot down:
_____
_____
_____
_____
_____
_____
_____

Honing your craft

I say this with all due respect for everyone out there: we all have to work at and hone our craft. Not for one season or for two but for a lifetime. Honing your craft is important no matter what industry you are in, no matter what role you are in. It is extremely important to make sure that you are consistently working at it, keeping up and even being at the forefront of new technological advancements and ensuring that you have your finger on the pulse of new changes and advancements, even before they are released to the market.

This means that you need to be dedicated. Why? Because it isn't easy to finish a week's worth of work, know that you have to go home and take care of your personal life, your home life, take care in keeping fit and still have time (or better yet, make time) for you to ensure that you are keeping up with all that requires to be done vis-a-vis the professional development landscape. It is so important that you spend time regularly visualizing the furthering of your career, whatever furthering your career means for you based on the promptings of the Holy Spirit.

Said differently, it is important for you to continue to visualize, pray and manifest as you continue on within your career. Some of the most successful people in the world are the ones who ensure that they consistently push themselves to do greater and go further.

An example of this is a family friend we have. He felt that he had worked hard enough in his career and was ready to stop or take a long break. He was still fairly young and his praying wife felt certain that he was not supposed to stop. They talked this out together respectfully and they both prayed about it. His wife used the 5-step method I have outlined and she felt led to pray for the Holy Spirit to provide her husband with some guidance, some motivation, a "push" if you will for what God wanted for her husband's life. What happened next is awesome: her husband was invited to a fishing trip with the guys and while this was during a time when their son was in the middle of a major sports tournament, she felt strongly that the Holy Spirit was encouraging her to support her husband going on the trip. She relented and he went on the trip. It changed his life. He reconnected with his old buddies, took risks on the trip, enjoyed working in nature and found that he really connected with nature. He came back from the weekend trip and told his wife that he felt tremendously motivated and excited to start a business of outdoor adventures. She was shocked since that wasn't exactly what she had in mind when she prayed for him to get motivated but it was a new direction the Holy Spirit was showing her to communicate and encourage her husband to take. After much deliberation and consideration between husband and wife, he now owns a thriving company that their son will be taking over one day, himself being a lover of sports and the outdoors and his wife works the front desk reception, greeting customers as they walk in and helping them find items they need for their outdoor sports and adventures.

Another example of this is the example of Martha. Martha is a very sweet and kind older lady. She was about 70 years old when I had the pleasure of making her acquaintance. She was a phenomenal painter but had never sold a painting. When I met her, she was wondering if she should continue painting or give it up since she wanted to make money with it but never had. I encouraged her to try this system and to see what the Holy Spirit was guiding her to do. When she closed her eyes, she saw a large downtown gallery and she saw some massive paintings hung up on the walls. They were much bigger than her own and so she was confused about what she was seeing, so we prayed about it together. We discovered that she was meant to expand her paintings and to tweak her current paintings just a bit. She had never painted that way so she was wondering what she should do. We prayed for the Holy Spirit to guide her paint brush. She began to paint in much broader strokes and in more muted colours. We felt led to a gallery downtown and even though she had never been to that gallery, she showed the owner a photo she had taken of her painting. Things lined up perfectly because the owner had said they were planning a show in a few months and he was looking for some bolder pieces. He invited her to have the pieces delivered to the gallery and she did. She has told her first paintings and she is now painting in the way that the Holy Spirit guides.

What am I saying? You never know which direction the Holy Spirit is going to take you but you need to be open to its promptings and you need to be open to how you're supposed to follow through. Ask questions of the Holy Spirit, probe, probe some more, ask further questions and know that you need to follow through on step 1 before step 2 may be revealed.

Focus on the image

When the Holy Spirit is giving you an image, make sure you focus on it. Focus carefully on all parts of it by looking and examining (yes, examining) each different aspect. Look carefully at the letters formed. For example, if you are visualizing an acceptance letter, see your name written carefully (is it in all caps, print or cursive?), see the positive words that you were hoping to see written actually written on the page, see the organization's logo and full name on the page. Take your time and let the close-up really sink in. Let yourself see the positive words that you wanted to see written on the page and carefully see your name written as the recipient of the good news.

I often visualize my email inbox with a new email from the person I was hoping to hear from, indicating the words "Offer" or the good news words I was hoping to read. I take my time and carefully look at each word written and I carefully examine the positive words. Yes, this means that I spend up to a full minute and sometimes longer seeing one word written that would indicate the good news I was hoping for.

Now, your good news correspondence may not (and likely will not look) in manifested reality look or be exactly as your vision was. But that's fine. The process still works. The manifestation is still taking place and is being created despite the actual reality maybe not looking exactly like that.

Don't miss out on your blessing because it didn't look exactly the way you saw it in your mind's eye.

Keep at it

Please remember to keep at this. If you don't see the good blessing manifesting right away, that's ok. It is still working. Keep working at it. This is a practice and it takes time.

The reason this book is called Manifest It....Now! is not because the manifestation will or has to happen now. It's a call to action to you to get started today (now, really) and to keep visualizing. It is only with consistent visualizing that you will really be able to manifest your God-given dreams and goals. It is only by consistently seeing the attainment of the goal in your mind's eye that it will become your lived reality.

> Remember: What you see in your mind consistently will eventually appear in your lived reality.

Praying for motivation & strength

I find it very important to also ask the Holy Spirit to give you the motivation and the strength to continue pushing yourself. If you are one of those people who finds it a bit challenging to keep on continuing, ask the Holy Spirit to guide you and show you how else you should push yourself. What else you should do and how so that you know that you are on the right track.

As humans, we can sometimes have a zeal for something and get excited, prompting us to start visualizing. Some people have the mentality that if it doesn't happen (manifest) right away, they will dump the practice. This is not a good idea. Please understand that it may likely take some time for things to manifest so you need to consistently give it the time, energy and dedication it requires. Doing a bit every day, day by day, week by week, month by month, will get you closer and closer and closer.

10

ENJOY THE MANIFESTATION AND GIVING GRATITUDE

When the manifestation does happen, enjoy it and do not forget to give thanks to God. When we really take the time to give thanks to God, He is more inclined to bring more good things to you. Said differently, if someone gives you something and you don't thank them for it, how likely are they to give you more good things? I don't know about you but I wouldn't appreciate that. God works the same way. Thank Him for what He has already done for you - this includes everything from being able to breathe to being able to speak and everything in-between. We cannot take for granted the basic functions that we are able to do because nothing is just given. Think of the many people out there who don't have the ability to breathe on their own, the many who cannot walk or are quadriplegic, who are wheelchair-bound, who are unable to write or who don't have all the necessary body parts, such as arms or a leg. We cannot take these things for granted and we have to remember to continually give thanks to God even for waking us up in the morning. This is such an important and powerful exercise and I suggest people do it regularly no matter what age or grade or activity level. Take stock of the good things in your life because being grateful for everything everyday is so important. You may wake up tomorrow and not have those same things anymore.

So, when we are asking God to cause something to manifest, we are asking Him to bring more good things into our lives. We are asking Him to continue adding to the pile that we already have, no matter what your pile already includes. It is so important to look around you and see not with an eye of greed or jealousy but to look around and see what others may not have that you do and how you can help them. Even if it's a simple act such as smiling at someone as you pass them by to let them know there are nice people out there, or helping a person in need with their groceries. I love seeing soup kitchens full of helping people because that means that those in need are getting the help they need. When you see a homeless person who is hungry, give them a prepaid gift card to a sandwich and coffee shop so they can (with dignity) go and get something nutritious and satisfying to eat. When you see an elderly person, help them by carrying something for them. All of these acts are important and are never wasted.

Take stock

 Before we begin with our list of ways we can express gratitude, let's take a moment and reflect on the good things we have. Write out your list here. Include everything.

Next, let's take some time to make a list of our thanks to people who do things for us each day, such as a parent, sibling, grandparent, friend, or other. If you write down a good thing that person has done or has given you, jot down next to it if you have thanked them. If you haven't, find a way that you would like to. Remember that it's never too late to thank a person.

_____
_____
_____
_____
_____
_____
_____

Expressing gratitude

Expressing gratitude and doing it in your own, personal way is so important. Most people enjoy receiving thanks for something so you will be making them happy by engaging in this.

Here are a few ways we can express gratitude. Remember that you can always put your special spin on these in any way that suits you. I have left extra space between ideas and on the bottom so you can put in your own spin on any of these:

- Write out your thanks in a journal

- Write the person a letter of thanks and send it by mail or by email

- Sing a song of praise & thanksgiving to the Lord for what He has done

- Write up a testimonial so that others can be encouraged and can see that God is still in the business of bringing miracles and consider posting it on a forum that is about testimonials

- When you go to Church on Sunday, remember to give thanks and praise Him

- Pay it forward and pray for what kindness you can do for another

- Increase your tithes payment and bless someone else

- If you write for or run a blog or website, share your news with others so that they too can see what you did and how you co-created with the Holy Spirit

- Spend time with the person by taking a walk together, going for coffee together, etc.

- Buy the person something simple but meaningful to them (ex. flowers, a nice gift, etc.)

- Still not sure what you should do? Pray about it. Ask the Holy Spirit to speak to you and to show you what that person might like. Remember that the Holy Spirit knows them better than you ever could.

Extra space:

Remember, giving thanks does not have to be expensive. It just has to be meaningful for you and for the person receiving it.

ABOUT THE AUTHOR

Dr. Christine Topjian is an Award-winning author of many books (and counting), an educator, an Executive Producer of film, television and new media works, ACTRA Performer and much more. She wears many hats in a day and enjoys practicing what she preaches.

She lives with her family in Thornhill, ON.

Catch up on more news, info and updates on Christine at drchristinetopjian.com. She is also on GoodReads as a verified author.

www.ingramcontent.com/pod-product-compliance
Lightning Source LLC
Chambersburg PA
CBHW071857160426
43209CB00005B/1086